Grow Bigger, Stronger and Last Longer Naturally:

The Ultimate Man's Guide to Stamina and Growth

Frank J. William

Copyright

Contents

4

Introduction

Men, if you have ever wished that you could last longer or be bigger below the belt, this is the book for you.

This book is divided into two sections, one for helping you gain endurance in bed and the other for helping you gain length and girth to your penis.

Say goodbye to low self-esteem and hello to the new, improved you.

When it comes to premature ejaculation, it is actually very common. However, tell any man who has ever had a problem with it that and it will not cheer them up overly much.

Men feel that they are expected to last long enough in bed to always give their partner an orgasm and that is just not the case.

No man is born with the ability to last tirelessly in bed, but they can learn how to increase their stamina and endurance so that they can last longer.

Sex will be better, for you and your partner.

Now, when it comes to penis size, there are no magic cures and nothing will give you fast results. As with anything, you will need to put time and effort into it but with those and patience, it is possible to gain length and girth.

Please remember that you need to follow the directions given for any exercises exactly, otherwise you can end up damaging your penis instead.

Penile Growth - The Basics

When it comes to size, it does matter. As a guy, when you know that you just do not measure up, it can affect your self-esteem, which can lead to further problems in the bedroom. This book is designed to help grow your penis, but slowly and safely over time.

You will need to do the exercises for several months before you see lasting results, but you will see results, it will just take time.

The reason it takes time is because the penis is rather delicate on the inside and through the application of gentle and constant exercises, you can achieve growth, safely.

The first thing that you will need to do is to measure yourself. Unless you measure yourself in the beginning and then again weekly, you will not know if the exercises are working right for you.

Many guys tend to measure their penis the wrong way, guys tend to measure their penis from the head of the penis to where it joins their body, and that is incorrect because your penis actually goes all the way to your pubic bone.

You will be measuring three things: your penis when flaccid, your penis when erect, and your girth. For this, you will need a ruler and a piece of string. Easy and simple!

To measure your flaccid penis, simply hold your penis straight out from your body, keeping it parallel to the ground and with a ruler, measure the length of the penis, the end of the ruler should be pressed into your pubic bone to get an accurate measurement.

To measure your erect penis, you do the same thing, only your penis needs to be fully erect and you will also need to hold it straight out from your body, keeping it parallel to the ground and measure in the same way that you measured your flaccid penis.

To measure your girth, your penis needs to be erect as well. Use a piece of string to wrap around the thickness of your penile shaft, about halfway down and then measure the string on the ruler to see what your girth, or thickness, of your erect penis is.

The exercises that will be in the later chapters of the book will require that you use a lubricant while performing them.

If you attempt to do these without a quality lubricant, you can end up causing major irritation, dryness and even chaffing to your penis.

Lubrication tends to wear off so while doing the exercises you will need to be mindful about reapplying whichever lubrication you have chosen to use.

You can purchase lubrication from any drug store or grocery store, silicon bases lubrications last longest and are the best but they are more expensive.

If you do not wish to buy lube, you can use lotion, but make sure that it is thick lotion and apply it frequently to keep from harming yourself.

Vaseline is also acceptable to use, but a bit messy and can cause stains on clothing so we really recommend that you stick with lube or lotion.

You might not think that pubic hair even factors into the equation about the length of your penis, but it does.

There are two reasons why it matters, first of all, when doing the exercises, unless you have shaved or trimmed your pubic hair, there is a very good chance that you will end up getting some caught in your hand and will end up pulling out hairs, which is never a pleasant experience.

The other reason is that pubic hair actually hides part of the length of your penis and so by getting rid of the pubic hair, your penis will naturally begin to look larger.

Bushy pubic hair can make your penis look almost half an inch shorter than it really is, so by shaving off your pubic hair, the full length of your penis can be seen easily.

Being overweight is another factor. Guys tend to accumulate fat in their stomachs, and when your stomach is fat, it causes an overhang affect and that diminishes the way your penis looks.

Your penis does not get smaller; it will just end up looking smaller because it is overshadowed by your belly.

Staying healthy is the first step in helping to keep yourself fit. The better condition that your body is in, the better it will respond to the exercises in this book.

The first thing that you should do is to ensure that you are always getting enough water to drink during the day.

When you are dehydrated, your blood does not circulate as well and without proper circulation, you will not get a very good erection because an erection is all about blood flow. Drink between 5-6 glasses of water a day, at a minimum to keep your body healthy.

Your diet should be a healthy and balanced diet, with less fast food and more freshly prepared meals at home. Lean proteins and fresh vegetables should be a good portion of your lunch and dinner meals.

When you eat healthy, you feel healthy, you look healthy, and that will go a long way towards helping to get your body in optimal shape and condition.

Your diet should contain fresh fruits, vegetables and lean protein, such as lean beef, turkey or chicken and you should limit the processed foods that you take.

Taking a multi-vitamin daily is also a good idea. Drop refined sugars, fast food, and foods that are laden with fat, such as processed snacks, bakery items, and fried foods.

If you are overweight, you need to increase your exercise level in order to lose weight and to ensure that your heart is healthy.

Thirty minutes of exercise three to four days a week will help you slim down, feel better, and help you with your stamina and endurance as well, because it all ties back into your heart health and your circulatory system.

Cardiovascular exercises are the proper way to get yourself into shape. All it takes is a little effort on your part.

Walking is the best exercise because it requires no special equipment and no gym membership; just start walking more and sitting less.

If you play sports, playing your sport of choice is a great way to boost your cardiovascular health; just half an hour of playing with friends will have your heart rate up and will help you burn calories.

Combining smart eating along with exercise is your ticket to health and will help your body be in the best shape that it can be in order for you to be able to begin your penile growth exercises.

Exercise Basics

This is the pre-exercise section of the book. First of all, let us say that if you suffer from any major medical conditions, especially heart conditions, circulatory conditions or any conditions that affect your skin, you should get medical clearance from your doctor to make sure that the exercises will not end up doing more harm than good.

If you are prone to rashes or if you have sensitive skin, these exercises might make the conditions worse because they are hands on exercises so always get clearance from your doctor.

When done properly, these exercises are safe. However, there is always a chance that if you are doing them incorrectly or too vigorously that you can end up bruising or chaffing your penis.

One of the signs that you need to look for is for small or medium bruise looking blue spots on your penis, which is a sign up bleeding beneath the skin, which is basically a bruise that forms from you being too rough or too vigorous with your exercising.

If you experience this, or chaffing, you need to take a few days off from your exercise regimen and let it heal and when you start up again, turn down the intensity a notch and you should be fine.

Before beginning the exercises in this book, you should always warm up. You warm up for other exercises, and these are no different.

If you fail to warm up, you can actually end up hurting yourself and then you will need to wait for your penis to heal before getting started again. Ignoring the warm up sessions can lead to bruises, torn skin and sores, which will be painful.

Your warm up session will help your body to get prepped for the exercises and it will prevent injuries from happening as well as to help make the exercises more effective. There are two ways you can warm up and both are equally effective.

You can use the hot wrap method to prepare your body for the exercises. By wrapping your penis and testicles in a hot towel, it will help prepare your body and your circulation system for the exercises that will follow.

Just be careful to not make it so hot that you scald or burn yourself. You will need either a washcloth or a small towel, such as a kitchen towel or hand towel.

You will need to run water until it is hot and completely soaked through and then wring it out so that you get all of the water out – if you leave much water in the towel and it is very hot, you are more likely to burn or scald yourself so always wring out all of the excess water; the goal is to have a hot but damp towel not a wet, hot towel.

Wrap the damp, hot towel around your testicles and penis, making sure that your entire penis is covered as well as the area at the base of your penis. Allow the damp towel to just stay wrapped until it starts to cool down to the touch.

As soon as it begins to cool, around two minutes, remove the towel or washcloth, run under hot water again wring it out again and wrap your penis and testicles again.

You will need to do this around four times total in order to properly warm up your body, especially your pelvic area and genitals for the exercises.

The other way that you can warm up is to take either a warm bath or a shower. The warmth helps the blood vessels circulate blood better and will help open them, increasing the blood flow near the surface of your skin.

It also helps loosen and relax the muscles in the area. Take a five-minute long warm bath or shower as your warm up before doing your exercises.

Jelqing

Jelqing is a well-known exercise that is very effective when it comes to helping to increase your penis girth and length. Jelqing has also been called penis milking, simply because of the action involved.

When done correctly and regularly, jelqing can increase your penis size safely and permanently. Your penis is full of blood vessels, capillaries, and spongy tissue that will fill with blood, causing an erection.

Jelqing is a way to increase penis length and girth by helping increase the blood flow into those blood vessels and capillaries.

When you increase the blood flow into the blood vessels and capillaries you are making more room for the blood to flow, not just that time, but in future times as well.

Jelqing helps your penis hold more blood, and that extra room for more blood adds length and girth. It may not be as obvious flaccid, but you will certainly notice the difference when you are erect.

It is not a speedy process so you will have to do the exercises regularly and keep at it.

There are a variety of pumps that do the same thing, they use suction to increase the blood flow to the penis, making it longer, however, that is a short lived effect and after a short period of time, the extra blood flow is gone, leaving you back at the same time. Jelqing is a permanent solution to extending your length.

This is no quick fix. It is a solution. When you reach the size that you desire, you can stop the exercises and your size will NOT revert to your original size, as it would with a penis pump.

The reason that these exercises are so well known is because they work, it is as simple as that. Remember to always warm up and to measure your penis once a week so you can track your progress.

There are many variations of jelqing but the main two categories are wet jelqing and dry jelqing. All variations of jelqing are based on these two types of jelqing.

Wet Jelqing

When you are practicing your wet jelqing exercises, you need to use lubrication. It is very important to use lubrication when doing wet jelqing and to make sure that you use enough lube or you can hurt yourself.

Keep the lubrication handy while doing the exercises because as soon as you feel that your penis is starting to get dry, add more lube.

It is always better to use more lube than necessary rather than not enough! Always precede your wet jelqing session with one of the two warm up ways that we discussed in the prior chapter.

Wet jelqing, also known as wet milking, is fairly easy. Use lube and be gentle with yourself as you do the exercises, you are trying to work with your penis, not punish it so follow the directions and be firm but gentle at the same time.

Wet jelqing requires that your penis is semi-erect. You cannot be fully erect and you cannot be flaccid. If you become fully erect during the exercise, you will need to stop to allow the erection to subside before beginning.

Do these exercises while fully erect can cause damage to the spongy tissues of your penis; you should only be half way erect, no more than that.

Start of using your left hand and touch the tip of your index finger to the tip of your thumb, forming the OK hand sign.

Grip the base of your penis with your circled thumb and finger so that your fingers are towards the top of your penis and your palm is facing outward and not towards your body.

Now, using the circle of your finger and thumb, move along the shaft of your penis, using a firm grip, but not so firm that it hurts or is uncomfortable, and slowly and steadily, while applying pressure, move your fingers to the tip of the penis.

If having your palm facing outward is too awkward of a position or if it is not easy for you to do, you can move your hand so that the fingers are below your penis and your palm is facing the body. It is whatever is easiest for you.

After going the length of your penis with your left hand, switch to your right hand and continue the exercise, the same way, only with your right hand instead.

Continue to switch hands and do this for at least fifteen minutes or longer; but as soon as it stops being comfortable, you should stop.

Dry Jelqing

The convenience about dry jelqing is that you do not need lube and therefore, there is less mess to clean up. Wet jelqing can be messy, lube is liquid and tends to splash and drip, and dry jelqing has none of the mess but still has the same effect.

It is a personal preference, many men prefer to do both; however, if you experience problems with dry jelqing, it is better to switch to wet jelqing, especially if your skin becomes irritated by dry jelqing.

Start with your warm up session, either damp, hot towels or a warm bath or shower to prepare for the exercise. Just like with wet jelqing, you need to maintain a semi-erection at about 50% hardness.

If you get more erect than that, you will need to stop and let it subside. We cannot stress enough that if you continue these exercises while erect, you can harm your penis.

The goal is not to orgasm and ejaculation is not the goal so when you begin to feel that you are getting more erect than 50%, stop and taking a break and continue when you are back at only being semi-erect. This is very important; as we have said, these exercises are safe, when done just as we describe.

Once again, use your finger and thumb to make the OK sign and then either with your palm towards your body or away from your body, hold your penis by the base and pull outward, such as if you were milking your penis.

Unlike the wet jelqing, you do not go to the tip of the penis, you only pull slightly, making sure to not slide your fingers over skin, you are pulling on the penis, not just moving your skin so have a firm grip and pull our firmly and only slightly pull forward on the penis.

Release your grip, return to the base of your penis, and repeat. Do this for a minimum of at least five minutes, and then begin again, but only slightly above the base of the penis and then with a firm grip, slowly and firmly pull on the penis.

Keep repeating this until you have worked your way to the tip of the penis. Then repeat with your right hand.

Stretching and the Warm Down

There are several products out there that promise to help stretch the penis, giving it more length; these products usually involve a weight of some sort being attached to the penis and then you allow it to hang, letting the weight and gravity do its job.

However, this is a great way to tear the inner workings of the penis, sprain it, or cause other injuries.

You can forego these often painful and expensive products and stretch your penis at home, safely, and comfortably.

You do not need to have lube for these exercises but some guys find that it is more comfortable to do with lube. It is totally up to you, it is your preference. If you start to hurt, you might want to try using a little lube, just to avoid chaffing or skin irritation.

It is very important that you do the stretching exercises only when your penis is flaccid. With Jelqing you needed to be half-way erect but for stretching, you need to be 100% flaccid.

If you attempt to do any of these exercises while you have an erection, even a slight one, you can damage the spongy tissue inside of your penis or cause injury to the capillaries or blood vessels leading to pain and bleeding under the skin.

If you begin to feel pain or discomfort while doing the exercises, do them with less pressure or just take a break and once again, do not attempt to continue them if you begin to get an erection, this is not a recommendation, it is vital to the health of your penis.

Here are a few stretching exercises that should be part of your daily routine, along with jelqing to help increase the length and girth of your penis.

Exercise 1

The first exercise that we are going to go over is the most common and one of the most useful and reliable ways to get results; it involves pulling on your penis and then twirling it.

How is twirling going to lengthen your penis? Well, when you twirl your penis, you are allowing it to move, using the weight of your penis to help keep the motion going, allowing it to stretch.

Just as with the jelqing exercises, you need to make an OK sign with your finger and thumb only instead of grasping your penis by the base, you grasp it with your finger and thumb just under the head of the penis.

Hold your penis firmly, but not so firm that you cut off the circulation. Pull your penis straight out in front of you, as far out as you can without it being uncomfortable or painful and then hold that position for about two to three minutes.

After two or three minutes, release your penis, but still hold onto it with your thumb and finger and then twirl your penis clockwise, do about 25 twirls to get the blood flow moving and then go back to holding the tip of your penis and pulling out from the head of the penis, only pull to the left this time and hold for two to three minutes again, and then twirl going counter-clockwise this time.

Repeat only pulling to the right, then down and then up and then go back to straight forward. Repeat the full circuit of directions at least five times, pausing to twirl between each time.

Exercise 2

In this exercise, you start off the same way, hold your flaccid penis just under the head of the penis and pull your penis straight forward and hold for about thirty seconds.

Still holding your penis stretched out with one hand, slap it against your right leg ten times and then ten times against the left leg.

Relax your penis slightly again and this time pull it to the right, hold for thirty seconds and then slap it ten times to your left leg and then to your right.

Repeat by pulling it to the left, then slapping it against each leg again.

Repeat this pattern several times.

Warm Down

Just like it was important to warm up prior to your stretching and exercising, it is equally important to have a warm down session afterwards.

The warm down tells your body and your penis that the exercises are over and it also helps with the results over the long term.

Since you are using your penis extensively, tugging, and pulling on it during the exercises, it will likely feel slightly sore, the skin of your penis can even be slightly irritated, and the warm down will help soothe the penis.

The first step is to gently massage your flaccid penis with your fingers for a few minutes. This will encourage the blood to flow and to circulate in the stretched tissues again.

After the massage, either do the hot wrap or the hot bath or shower that we went over in the warm up session section. It does not matter which you choose but you need to do one or the other to help your penis recover and to prevent any injuries.

The warm up and warm down are very important so never forget to do them. If you have not got the time to warm up, exercise and stretch and then warm down, skip your session for the day or do it when you have more time during that day.

Additional Exercises

Several other exercises can be used to help improve the length and girth of your penis. You can choose to do any or all of these additional exercises, simply do them along with your other exercises or in place of but always do the warm up and the warm down.

You can make your own exercise plan, rotating what exercises you do daily to give yourself some variety and avoid getting bored with the exercises.

Remember, you will need to do these daily, or near daily for months to see any significant growth, but you will see growth. You just have to stick with it.

Additional Exercise 1

Your penis needs to be in a flaccid state. Take a firm grip on your penis, just below the head of your penis, but not hard enough to cut off your circulation or to be painful.

Pull your penis out in front of you, as far as you comfortably can and hold this stretched position for a good thirty seconds and then release your penis and allow it to rest for about fifteen seconds and then repeat.

Continue doing this until you have accumulated about 15 minutes of total time with your penis stretched out.

Additional Exercise 2

This exercise begins with your penis flaccid and then ends with it erect. Because it is easier to damage your penis when erect, you need to follow the directions exactly how they are listed to avoid injury.

With your penis in the flaccid state, take hold of it with your right hand, just below the head of the penis and pull away from your body, holding for twenty seconds and then relaxing briefly, then pulling straight out again, holding for twenty seconds. Do this a total of ten times.

Repeat this only pulling to the left, then the right, and then down.

Now, give yourself an erection, you can either stroke your penis or rub the head of the penis until you are erect; however, you prefer to do it, but you need to be fully erect to complete the exercise.

Use your thumb and finger to make the OK sign again and circle the base of your penis. You can have your palm facing out or facing your body, it does not matter which, however is more comfortable for you. Pull forward about an inch to a half inch and then relax. Do this about fifteen times.

Switch to holding your penis by just below the head of the erect penis and then pull your penis to the left while rotating it in small circles.

Do this fifteen times and then pull to the left while making small circles with your penis and do this fifteen times.

Once again holding your penis by the base, pull out from the base of the erect penis and slap it against your right inner thigh fifteen times and then to the left fifteen times.

Additional Exercise 3

This is an exercise that is useful for enlarging the glans of the penis. The glans is the head of the penis and the size of that can also be increased through exercise.

If you are just looking for girth and length and have no interest in increasing the size of the head of your penis, then just skip this exercise.

For this exercise, you will need to have lubrication so either lotion or lube will work. You need to get yourself into a semi-hard state or about 50% erect.

Just like with the jelqing, if you find yourself getting more than 50% erect then you need to stop the exercise and wait for the erection to lessen.

Once again, using your thumb and finger, make the OK sign and circle the base of your penis, with firm pressure. Take your other hand and hold your penis just above your other hand. You will have both hands on your lubricated penis at this point, with one hand just above the other, both hands in the OK formation, fingertip to thumb tip.

Using the same forward motion as with the wet jelqing technique, move both hands firmly forward, towards the head of your penis and stop when your top hand is just at the bottom of the head of your penis.

Release your top hand, the hand that is closest to the head of your penis and then grip the base of your penis with that hand, with your thumb and finger, just like before.

Keep the other hand at the head of the penis, it was the hand that was on the base of your penis, and now it is at the head of your penis.

Now, slide the hand that is at the base of your penis up to the head of your penis, so that it is just below your other hand. Release the hand at the head of the penis and then circle your penis at the base again and move that hand firmly up the shaft of the penis, until it is just below the hand already at the head of your penis.

It might take you a minute to get the rhythm going, but you will continue to do that, keeping one hand constantly in motion for at least two minutes.

The PC Muscle

We will use this chapter to segue into the second half of the book, which will focus on fixing premature ejaculation.

The PC muscles are not only involved in ejaculation control, endurance, and stamina, but when you exercise the muscles, it will help increase the size of your penis by adding muscle and strengthening the muscles.

The PC muscle is very important, because it will also help with your prostrate by keeping it healthy and it can help with incontinence.

In fact, these exercises are similar to the exercises used by women to regain pelvis muscle strength after childbirth.

Exercising your PC muscles will help you gain control of your erections and by strengthening the muscles that can control your penis, it will help your penis in terms of size as well.

The PC muscle will not only help you perform better but it will help you look better as well, which is why it helps both parts of your problem.

First of all, you need to know where your PC muscle is located. You have already used this muscle often; you probably just have not known what it is called. The PC muscle is the muscle that runs between your scrotum and your anus.

You use the muscle when you stop your urination flow mid-stream and it is the same muscle that you use to move your penis when you have an erection, without your hands of course.

Since you are probably not used to working these muscles very much, take the exercises slowly, building up your endurance.

Start with shorter sessions and then build up to longer ones as you build up your endurance and feel the muscle begin to strengthen.

Exercise 1

This is a very basic exercise and it focuses on contracting and then relaxing the PC muscle. Simply contract the muscle and then the relax it.

Do not hold the PC muscle tense, just contract and relax. Try to do fifteen of these at first but if you can do more, then do more, but stay within your comfort zone, especially because you are not used to these.

After doing the first set give yourself a three-minute rest and now you are going to do the same thing, contract and release, but in clusters of three, holding each contraction for three seconds.

Contract the PC muscle, hold for three seconds and then release, contract again and hold for three seconds and then release and then contract again, hold for three seconds and then release and then rest for about fifteen seconds and do another cluster of three.

Do this for a minimum of fifteen times.

When doing a set of fifteen becomes too easy, add five more contractions. Ideally, every three or four days you should be increasing the amount of contractions that you are doing daily until you are able to do sets of thirty at a time, with a two minute break in-between.

Just keep increasing the number of contractions per set and the length of time that you can hold each contraction. The good thing about these exercises is that you can do them anywhere and nobody will be able to tell.

You can do them clothed while at home or at work, which makes them the ultimate exercise. You can do several sets per day, taking a long rest in between sets.

You can add breathing techniques to the exercise, the benefit of adding breathing exercises is that it allows you help hold the muscles tense for longer than just three seconds.

To synch your breathing along with the contracting and releasing of your PC muscle, you will first need to get your breathing into a nice, steady rhythm.

Your breathing should be slow and deep, as if you are fully relaxed.

Now, with your breathing remaining steady and slow, begin to contract the PC muscle and hold it as tight as you possibly can and when you have gotten it as tense as you possibly can, hold the contraction and then count to twenty, keeping your breathing slow , even and deep.

Do not hold your breath while holding the contraction. After you release the contraction, continue to breathe and allow yourself to rest for about thirty seconds.

Repeat this at least five times. As you build up your endurance and stamina, you can hold the contraction for long periods of time and you can repeat it for more than five times. Try to hold the contraction for at least a minute.

Your sex life will begin to improve with these exercises, you will begin to see a vast improvement in your performance, and more importantly, your partner will see a difference and feel the difference!

Take your time building up your PC muscle, if you try to push yourself and overdo it, you can actually strain or pull the muscle, which will not be very comfortable so if your body tells you that you are pushing too much, dial it back and give it a rest.

Variation Exercise 1

In this exercise, you will follow the basic directions and the goal is to have the contractions increase in intensity. By intensity, we mean the strength of the contraction.

Start off with a light contraction of the PC muscle, hold it for a few seconds, and then relax. Contract the muscle again, only contract it just a little bit harder, hold it for a few seconds, and then relax.

Keep building up the intensity of the contractions, and each time you only need to make the contraction slightly more intense by squeezing the muscle just a little tighter each time and hold it for a few seconds longer.

Continue to do this until you are squeezing the PC muscle as tightly as you can, and you cannot squeeze it any more; hold it at that maximum tensed position for at least five seconds and then release.

Take a minute to relax and then begin the process all over. Remember to slowly increase the tension in the contraction, you are going to try to get to your maximum contraction strength over a span of four or five contractions not just one or two.

Repeat sets of these for about 10 minutes or until you begin to have trouble holding the contraction.

Variation Exercise 2

This is similar to the first variation exercise, only
instead of contracting the muscle slightly, holding
it, releasing it and then repeating with each
contraction getting stronger you will begin with a
light contraction but instead of holding it and
releasing it, you will keep the muscle contracted
lightly and then tense it slightly more and hold it
and then slightly more, and hold it and so forth until
you cannot tense the muscle any more.

When you have the muscle tensed as much as it
possibly can be, hold it for at least twenty to thirty
seconds and then relax.

Premature Ejaculation Basics

Premature ejaculation is more common than you probably think and trust us when we say that you are not alone.

It is estimated that somewhere around 30% of the male population suffers from premature ejaculation. Even for those who do not have premature ejaculation, many men still wish that they could last longer in bed than they do.

In fact, when asked what they could change about their love life, many men have said that they wish that they could last longer in bed.

Premature ejaculation can cause serious self-esteem issues and it can have a negative effect on a man's ego. It can cause problems with their partner and it can actually cause enough stress and tension that a relationship can actually end up terminating over it.

Premature ejaculation is just what it sounds like it means, it is when the male ejaculates too quickly, usually within a matter of a minute or two.

It happens to everybody at some point or another but when it becomes a lasting and lingering problem, that is when it begins to cause problems and that is where this book will help you.

Many men feel that they are not lasting as long as they could or that they need to in order to please their partner. Even if they are not ejaculating prematurely, they may be ejaculating sooner than their partner may.

This book will help you be able to last longer. It is a simple fact that women take longer to get to their climax stage. Even if you last longer than average in bed, if you finish before your partner, then it can still be viewed as a problem.

Even if the woman does not make an issue out of it, men often do because their ability to satisfy their partner can impact their partner.

The average male only lasts between three to six minutes in bed. In fact, over half of the male population ejaculates within two to three minutes after penetration. The problem arises because it takes the average woman almost fifteen minutes to reach their climax.

If the average woman takes fifteen minutes and the average man takes only two, which is a lot of women who are not getting satisfied.

You may have thought that you were one of a few with this problem, but in fact, you are one of many, in fact, you are in the majority, not the minority!

Knowing that does not make you feel any better but this will, the problem is fixable and you can train yourself to last longer when it comes to sex.

Remember, the goal is not just to last longer, but to satisfy your partner so that she orgasms.

When you work on lasting longer in bed and at the same time, knowing how to please her so she is able to climax faster means that you both win.

Keep in mind that sex involves much more than just penetration; it includes oral sex, foreplay, even erotic massage, and penetration.

What are some of the common causes for premature ejaculation?

Genetics - the fact is that if your DNA is coded to have you climax quickly, you end up climaxing quickly. Keep in mind that humans are the only mammals that have sex for pleasure; in nature, mammals are designed to ejaculate quickly and humans are no different. Our DNA tells us that sex is for reproductive reasons only and we have to try to overcome that.

Masturbation - when men masturbate, they tend to focus on trying to ejaculate quickly, especially when they hit puberty and the rush of hormones hit. Masturbation is usually done quickly and very much in secret and it is actually training your body to go ahead and climax as quickly as you can. After so many years of this, our bodies are used to it and it becomes a hard habit to break.

Anxiety and stress - Stress and anxiety takes a huge toll on the human body. It keeps us from performing at our peak and our bedroom performance is no different. If you suffer from performance anxiety, it makes it even worse. The more you worry about if you will perform better the worse your performance will end up being! You need to just calm your mind and stop worrying about your performance and just let it happen.

Weak PC muscles - we went over this the prior chapter, but your PC muscles greatly affect your performance

Positions - some positions end up putting more pressure on your pelvic muscles than others and that can actually contribute to you climaxing earlier.

Lifestyle - things such as being inactive and eating high calorie and fatty foods can cause premature ejaculation.

You can condition your body to overcome premature ejaculation. All of the above factors can be overcome with practice.

Anybody who has ever watched porn can tell you that the male performers last for a long time, much longer than you can. They are not born with that ability, they learn to do it, and you can learn as well.

Ignore the wealth of products that are to be found on the shelves of many stores. There are no creams, sprays, or pills that will give you endurance and the ability to last longer in bed.

The sprays and creams have ingredients that desensitize you, so that you last longer because you can feel less!

Why buy a product that takes away the feeling of sex? It makes no sense but it is the sacrifice that many men make in order to please their partner.

There is no quick fix for premature ejaculation but there is a fix. Your sex life will be transformed and this book is the first step.

The Mental Factor

No doubt, you have heard the phrase, "it is all in your head" before and it actually hold true to this scenario as well.

Our brains are the control center for our entire body, including the penis and so a big factor in not lasting as long as we want in bed comes from how we think about sex.

Change your thinking and change your sex life, for the better.

How important is your thinking when it comes to helping with premature ejaculation? How about over half of it can be fixed by changing your thinking, as a matter of fact, almost 70-75% of the premature ejaculation issues are caused by your brain, from your thinking and not from a physical source at all!

The cortex is the part of the brain that controls stimulation and excitement, and therefore, ejaculation. When something begins to arouse you, your cortex perks up and takes notice and it is what tells your body to react physically.

Knowing that your mind exerts influence over your body can help a large amount of your problems because you will be able to use it to your advantage!

If you ejaculate too fast because you get too excited, learning to calm down your cortex will help delay your orgasm and your ejaculation; it works both ways.

When you are having sex, it feels good. Of course, it feels good, that is why we have sex, right! As we have sex, our senses are bombarding us, and it can actually overload us, contributing to the problem of premature ejaculation.

As males, sometimes we tend to treat sex like a race, thinking that the only part that matters is the actual intercourse and that we must hurry up and get there, and by the time that we rush through foreplay and then have sex, we have been looking forward to it so much that our cortex literally overloads with pleasure and we climax quickly.

Change your thinking so that you are not focused on intercourse as the goal, but rather the entire sexual experience.

Enjoy it from start to finish, take your time, and make it sensual and erotic, focusing on each thing that you are doing and focusing less on getting foreplay out of the way so you can have sex.

Make pleasing your partner your priority and not pleasing yourself. Why? Because you will still end up climaxing, only it will not be so early. Sex might be good now, but it can be so much better and this will make it better for you both.

Remember, women take nearly fifteen minutes to get to the climax stage and men only need a fraction of that so stop rushing towards intercourse.

Make foreplay fun. Be erotic and sensual and make her climax before you even have intercourse. When you are focusing on her pleasure, your brain is not so focused on the act of intercourse and when you do have intercourse, it will last longer.

Do not try distraction tricks. No thinking about sports or anything visually unappealing because that just takes the pleasure and the fun away from sex.

Focus on giving her an orgasm. Focus on the curves of her body and how to tease pleasure from them for her and keep your mind on that. Do not distract yourself from sex, which takes away so much of the pleasure and makes it seem like a chore, not something fun.

Try thinking positively about your premature ejaculation; use the power of visualization to see yourself lasting longer in bed. Do not just wish for it to happen but visualize it happening. Visualize this often and it will come true.

Keep your thoughts positive. Negative self-talk only leads to lower esteem and that can be a vicious cycle to climb out of so when you find yourself thinking that you cannot last as long as you want, erase that thought from your mind right away.

Do not let the negative thoughts dwell in your head because once you let them take root, they will grow and it will be even harder to get rid of them.

Strike those negative thoughts out as soon as you have them and replace it with a positive thought. Instead of thinking that you will disappoint your partner tonight, think that you will please your partner tonight.

Always, always keep a positive outlook and mental attitude.

To last longer in bed you need to learn to control your arousal building. Once you are aroused past a certain state, climax cannot be delayed and it will happen. If you learn to slow down your arousal so that you do not get overly aroused from the start, you can learn to last longer in bed.

When you find yourself about to have sex after a satisfying round of foreplay and you find yourself quickly becoming aroused to the point where you are about to end up climaxing and it is too soon, change up the sex to be slightly less intense.

Slow down your speed, do not penetrate her as deeply, or even switch to a position that you do not enjoy quite as much; this will continue to allow your arousal to build but it will build up slower, allowing you to last longer in bed, which is the goal.

You can even start and stop sex, continue with some foreplay and then continue having sex. Trust us, your partner will not complain at the attention or the pleasure that you will give her so it is a win-win situation no matter how you look at it.

You can help to control your arousal by controlling your sex. When you feel yourself getting aroused too quickly, slow down your breathing and you will actually slow down your rate of arousal as well.

As you breathe, focus on filling your belly with air and not your lungs and you want your shoulders to be still.

Most of us breathe all wrong, using only the top part of our lungs and our chest to breathe, which makes our shoulders hitch up and down as we inhale and exhale but when we breathe the correct way, our shoulders are still, and our abdomen rises and falls instead.

Takes long slow breaths, from your stomach and then let it out. Whenever you need to slow your arousal, just shift part of your mental attention to your breathing, it works!

The Physical Factor

The natural progression from using your mind to controlling your body is to include the physical factor, things that you can physically do to help with premature ejaculation.

You can condition your body to not climax as quickly and you can build up your endurance and your sexual stamina this way but it requires a lot of self-knowledge.

Make this fun, include your partner, and turn this into something fun, erotic, and sensual.

We have already gone into the PC muscles. Those are the muscles that control your ejaculation and so when you can strengthen them, you are better able to physically hold off your ejaculation by tensing them, holding off on your climax.

You should use the exercises that are in The PC Muscle chapter daily to build up your PC muscles, giving you better control and endurance.

We taught you how to exercise the PC muscles but now we will go over how to use them to ward off a climax that is coming sooner than you want it to.

For this exercise, you need to get yourself to the point of almost reaching orgasm. Remember how we mentioned how masturbating quickly can lead to premature ejaculation, well because of that, you are not trying to race yourself to climax.

If you are masturbating, take your time at it, because otherwise you are still conditioning yourself to climax quickly. You can bring yourself to almost a climax with your partner as well.

Just as long as you get yourself right to the point of nearly climaxing and then when you only a few seconds away, tense up your PC muscles as tight as you can and hold it. Do not hold your breath, continue to breathe but keep your PC muscle flexed and tense.

Hold you PC muscles until you feel your arousal being to fade slightly so that you are able to relax your PC muscle and not ejaculate upon release.

Learning the timing to this will take time and practice, so do not get discouraged if it takes you many times to get the timing of this down correctly.

You can actually use masturbation as a tool to help you build your stamina as well. You can get yourself used to hitting a certain level of pleasure and then stopping.

The idea is to get used to being able to withstand the pleasure for longer and longer periods without getting to the point where ejaculation and climax is a certainty.

Find a comfortable spot, someplace where you feel free and comfortable to be able to masturbate without being disturbed, so turn off your cell and turn off the TV. This exercise requires just you and your sensations.

Begin to masturbate but do so slowly. Taking note of the feelings that you are producing in your own body and enjoy them.

Focus on how good it feels, you are trying to also get your mind to focus on the here and now and not the thought of climax.

Slowly continue to build up your arousal until you are about 40% towards climaxing. Stop masturbating, let your hands rest in your lap or off to your sides and just let your body relax and let your mind just feel the sensations of your arousal and how it is fading.

Take a few deep breaths, just like we outlined in the prior chapter, from your belly and not your chest.

When you feel that you are back down to only being at a 20% arousal state, begin to masturbate again, still going slowly so that you are able to savor the sensations.

This is not only getting you used to higher levels of stimulation but you are conditioning your mind that what leads up to climax is just as important as climax itself as well.

Continue until you feel that you are about 60% of the way toward climaxing and then once again stop masturbating, breathe deeply from your belly and relax your body until you are back at 20% aroused.

Continue to masturbate again until you reach 80% of the way to climax and then stop, breathe deeply, and then relax until your arousal drops back to 20%.

Continue again until you are at 90% and then stop, breathe deeply, then relax until your arousal drops to 20%, and then repeat, until you finally end up climaxing.

Here is another exercise for you to do; this will help you to build up your endurance.

In the prior exercise, you allowed your arousal to drop down to 20% before bringing it back up, which means that you were becoming erect and then back to a near flaccid state repeatedly.

This exercise is designed to be done without you losing your erection

Begin to masturbate and do so until you are about 60% aroused and once you reach that 60% mark, stop masturbating, and allow your arousal to drop to 40%, you should still be erect at 40%.

Do this five times, allow yourself to get to 60% and then drop back to 40%.

The sixth time you begin to masturbate, get yourself to the 80% arousal point and then drop it back down to 60%. Do this five times.

Repeat again, only going to 90% aroused and then dropping to 70%.

Keep repeating at 90%/70% and continue to do so until you climax. With practice, you should be able to get yourself to at least thirty minutes with an erection before you climax.

When you reach the thirty minute mark, begin all over again, only use lubrication, this will more closely match the feel of actual sex.

Additional Thoughts on Premature Ejaculation

We have gone over how your thinking can affect your premature ejaculation and have gone over how you can condition your body to overcome your tendency to ejaculate too soon and this chapter covers pretty much everything else that you need to know when it comes to premature ejaculation and pleasing your partner.

We mentioned it briefly in a prior chapter, but the position that you are having sex in can make you more prone to ejaculating quicker.

That does not mean that you should avoid that position. It just means that you should limit your use of that position. For example, use that position for a bit, then stop and switch to a different position for a while.

Switching up positions is not only fun, but also during those few seconds where and your partner are getting into a new position it will act as a mini-cool down for your arousal, helping you to last longer that way.

The missionary position, the most popular position for sex is actually the position that is the most prone to making you ejaculate before you want to.

In the missionary position, your body weight on your arms and legs will end up working against you, causing you to come too soon simply because of the tension that it places on those muscles and because it puts more friction on your penis.

Instead of the missionary position, use the cowgirl. This position takes pressure off of the most sensitive part of your penis, which is the frenulum and is right underneath the head of your penis on the bottom.

When you use the missionary position, you are putting a lot of friction on that part of the penis, which makes you ejaculate quicker and the cowgirl position – where the girl is on top – does not put as much pressure on that part of your penis, allowing you to last longer.

With the woman on top and facing you, you are thrusting up into her, causing less friction on your penis and you will be able to last longer.

Additionally, you are taking pressure off of your legs and arms, which means less pressure on your pelvis muscles, which is another factor in causing you to ejaculate prematurely.

An alternative of this is the reverse cowgirl, where your partner is on top of you but facing away from you.

Another position that works really well because it also does not put pressure on your arms and legs is the side position, also called spooning. You and your partner both lie on your sides and she will have your back up against your chest. You will both need to bend your legs and her hips should be right at your groin so that you can penetrate her.

This side-by-side position gives you complete control over how deep you penetrate her and lets you set the pace and so when you begin to feel like you are becoming aroused too quickly, you can simply slow down and then speed back up again when you feel like it.

This position is very erotic and sensual because of the close nature of the position.

Now that you know a few other positions that work well to keep your ejaculation delayed, you can keep switching positions, so that you rotate them.

As previously stated, just changing out your position will give you a mini-recharge and will help you last longer.

Something else that we mentioned was that most men feel that they are ejaculating prematurely because they are climaxing before their partner. If they make their partner's orgasm a priority, then this will no longer be a factor anymore.

Being skilled at oral sex and foreplay is a great way to help her achieve her climax quicker. Men sometimes tend to go straight for the vagina and then they wonder why they climaxed but their partner did not.

Foreplay is an art form and you need to become a master.

Turn sex into a full-bodied experience. Engage her entire body, from nibbling her ears to running your fingers lightly over her body, all over.

Caress her and kiss her all over. The more stimulation to her that you provide during foreplay, the quicker she will build up her own arousal and the quicker she will be able to climax.

Learn to use your mouth and your fingers to dial into her pleasure zones and to bring her to orgasm and then you can have sex, with the tips that we have gone over in the book already, you will be a master lover at this point, lasting longer than ever before and the attention that you show her prior to you climaxing will be like none other.

Conclusion

The male ego is so closely related our ability to perform up to our own standards in the bedroom that it can greatly affect us when we are not performing up to par.

The problem is, the person who we are disappointing is not our partners, but we end up feeling as if we have, no matter what they say.

If a male feels inadequate, it will be hard for him to overcome that feeling, no matter what assurances his partner gives him. The fact is that not all men are created equal and it is natural to want to be bigger and last longer in bed.

If men were not so worried about their penis size and their ability to last longer during sex, there would not be such a huge market for products that are designed to help one or the other.

Men do worry and all too often they waste so much money on products and gimmicks that never end up working, leaving them feeling even more let down than before.

Increasing your penis size is nothing more than building up muscle and stretching it to allow for more room for the blood to flow. You just have to be patient and work with your penis but you will see results over time.

Just remember to follow the directions exactly as we have them and to always warm up then have your sessions and then warm down. Never stretch or do the penile growth exercises without a warm up or the warm down.

When it comes to premature ejaculation, learning to exercise control of your PC muscle is only the first step towards being able to last longer in bed.

Our series of exercises is designed to increase your arousal periods and help you last longer, which means that you will have even more time to enjoy sex.

www.ingramcontent.com/pod-product-compliance
Lightning Source LLC
Chambersburg PA
CBHW020408290526
45785CB00005B/2470

* 9 7 8 1 3 0 4 2 7 9 9 5 8 *